Periodontal diseases affect millions of people. These diseases start very early in life and cause the loss of more teeth than all other reasons combined. In the early stages, periodontal diseases are silent infections. In most cases you are not aware that problems exist until the disease is quite advanced.

- What are periodontal diseases?
- Who gets them?
- How do they start?
- Can you prevent them?
- Can they be successfully treated once they start?

This booklet answers these questions.

This publication explains general principles. There are individual exceptions. Your own dentist's advice is the best advice you can get.

PART I

PART I gives you general information about periodontal diseases: the signs, the causes, and what you and your dentist can do to prevent periodontal diseases or arrest disease that has already started.

INTRODUCTION

Each tooth consists of two parts: the *crown* and the *root(s)*.

Normally, only the crown is visible in the mouth. The roots anchor the tooth in the bone.

The *gums* are a specialized type of skin that surrounds the teeth and covers the bone holding the teeth.

Each front tooth has one root. Back teeth have one, two, or three roots.

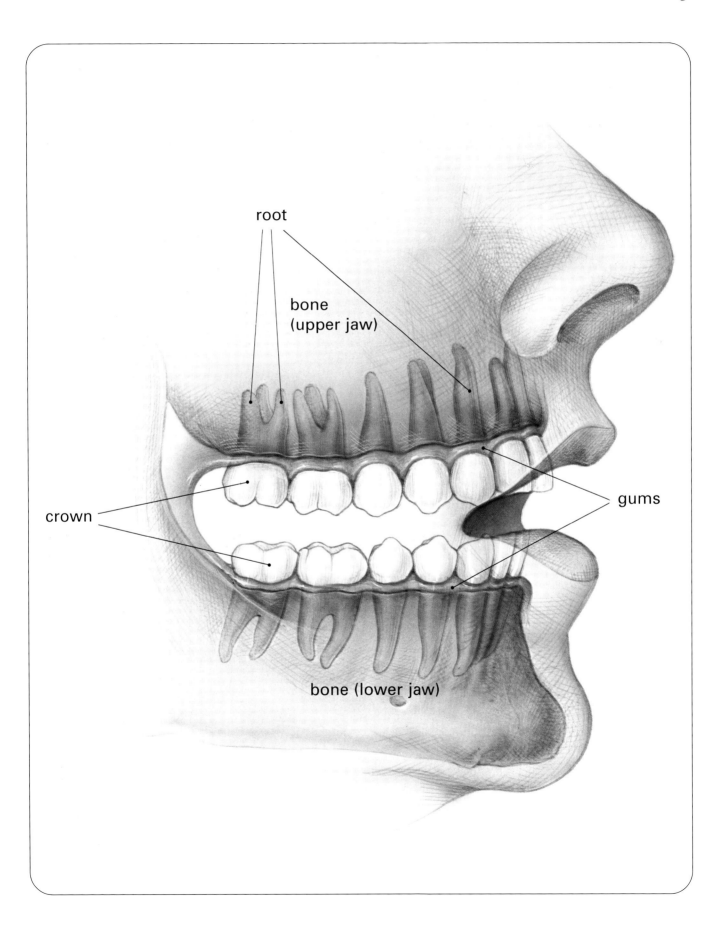

root

bone
(upper jaw)

gums

crown

bone (lower jaw)

NORMAL GUMS

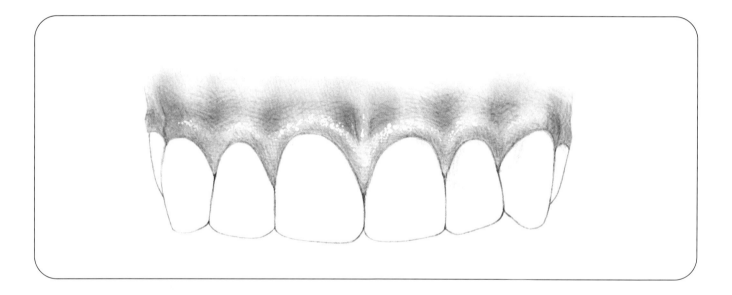

This diagram shows the gums of a person who has a light com-plexion. People with dark skin normally have gums that are quite a bit darker.

INFECTED GUMS

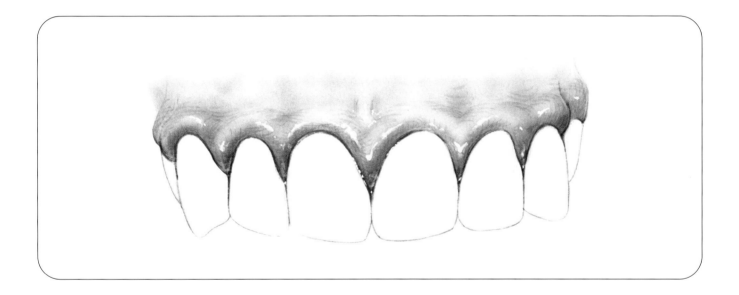

Sometimes, gums that are infected look like this.

But

Many people who have gum infections, even in advanced stages, may have gums that look essentially normal. That is why only a thorough examination by a dental professional can detect most gum problems.

STAGES OF PERIODONTAL DISEASES

Periodontal diseases can be divided into two stages:

• Gingivitis
• Periodontitis

GINGIVITIS

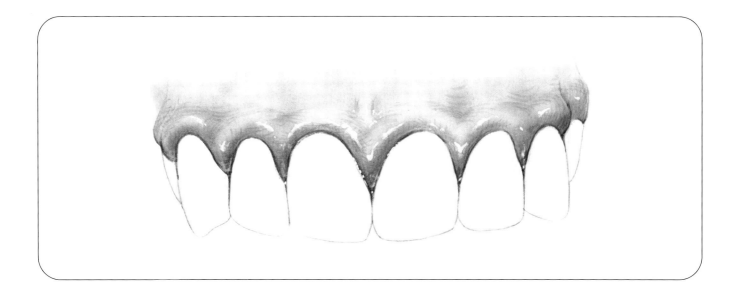

Gingivitis is a superficial infection that is limited to the gum tissue and does not yet affect the underlying bone. The gums may look normal, but may have some of the following signs:

1. Redness and puffiness
2. Bleeding when brushed
3. Bad odor

PERIODONTITIS

When the infection spreads from the gum to the underlying bone, it is termed *periodontitis* (once called *pyorrhea*). In this stage, bone that supports the teeth is lost. There are several types of periodontitis, some more aggressive than others. If periodontitis is untreated, tooth loss can occur.

In some cases the gums appear red and swollen, and other signs may warn you of trouble:

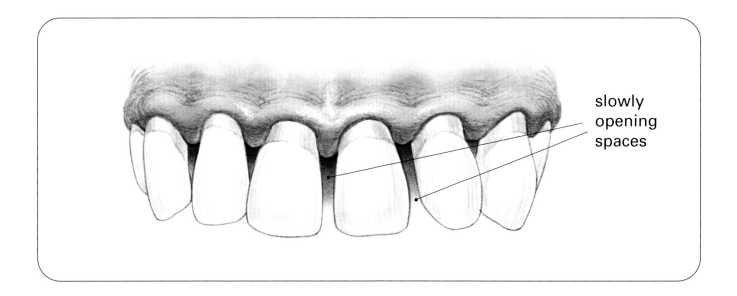

slowly
opening
spaces

1. *Spaces* begin to appear between the teeth. This can be a sign of an advanced problem.

2. *Loosening* of one or more of the teeth. This is almost always a sign of severe bone loss.

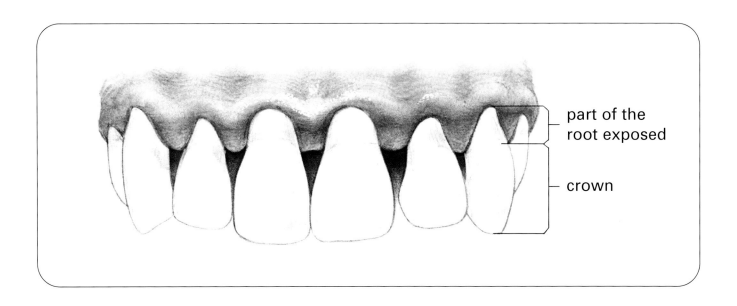

part of the root exposed

crown

3. *Receding gums.* Periodontal diseases may cause gums to shrink away from the crown and expose some of the root. This makes the teeth look longer. Gum recession is not normal at any stage.

4. *Vague aching, itching, or other discomfort of the gums.*

Periodontal diseases are almost always painless, and only rarely do you notice changes, especially in the early stages. Therefore, you probably will not notice gum puffiness or pay attention to occasional bleeding when you brush. Or you may think that the longer look of your teeth is normal for your age. *But the fact is, four out of five teenagers and adults have periodontal disease, and most don't know it.* That is why people lose more teeth from periodontal diseases than from all other reasons combined.

But the good news is that *most periodontal diseases can be prevented or, if already started, can be treated.* This is particularly true *if action is taken in the early stages of disease.*

PLAQUE IS THE PRIMARY CAUSE
OF PERIODONTAL INFECTION

Every day a sticky, almost invisible film forms on the teeth. This film is *plaque*,* a continually spreading mass of disease-causing bacteria and their waste products. Plaque grows on the teeth and down into the crevice between the gum and tooth. When the underlying bone is lost, this crevice deepens and is called a *pocket*.

In very large amounts, plaque can be seen or can be felt with the tongue as a fuzzy, unclean coating on the teeth.

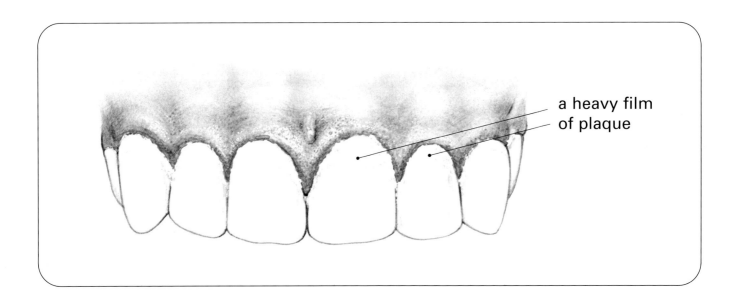

a heavy film
of plaque

*Pronounced "plack."

The bacteria of plaque produce *toxins* (poisons) that damage the gums and underlying bone.

PLAQUE BECOMES CALCULUS

If you do not completely remove plaque every day by toothbrushing and flossing, it leads to the formation of *calculus* ("tartar"), a stony crust with a pitted, rough surface.

It takes only a little more than a day for any plaque left on your teeth to turn into calculus.

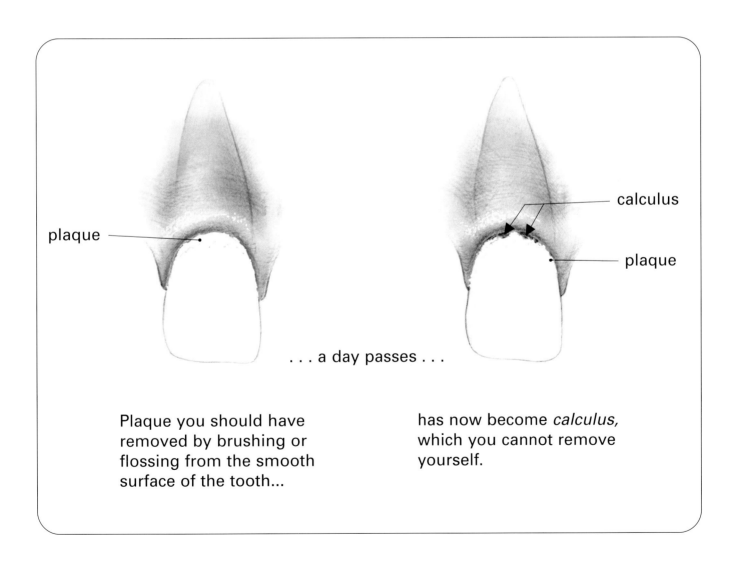

plaque

. . . a day passes . . .

calculus

plaque

Plaque you should have removed by brushing or flossing from the smooth surface of the tooth...

has now become *calculus,* which you cannot remove yourself.

You can't remove calculus yourself. It clings to the teeth with such force that only a dentist or hygienist can remove it.

It is possible to see calculus that forms *above* the gums. It appears as a brownish or black deposit around the necks of the teeth. However, *it is the hidden calculus under the gums* that does the most harm.

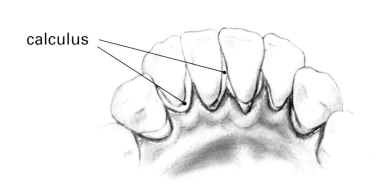

calculus

backs of lower front teeth, just in front of the tongue, a common place to see calculus buildup

Calculus greatly complicates the problem of preventing periodontal diseases. Each day's new plaque embeds itself in the rough surface of calculus in such a way that *no toothbrush, or dental floss, or any other home dental device can ever remove it!*

Thus, all calculus will always have plaque embedded on its surface. And all plaque is capable of starting or worsening periodontal diseases.

It is very important that you never let calculus get a start. Floss and brush away plaque every day. Never let plaque remain long enough to become calculus.

To sum up oral hygiene:

• YOU CAN remove sticky plaque from your teeth.

• YOU CAN'T safely remove calculus or the plaque that forms on the surface of calculus, especially below the gums.

PLAQUE TOXINS DESTROY BONE

The toxins produced by the bacteria in plaque not only infect the gum, but also *destroy the underlying bone that supports the teeth.*

As the gum infection continues, so does the bone destruction, usually without any symptoms, especially in the early stages of the disease.

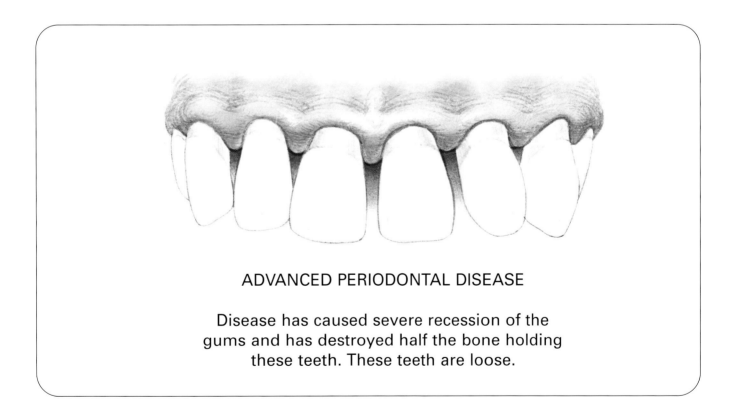

ADVANCED PERIODONTAL DISEASE

Disease has caused severe recession of the gums and has destroyed half the bone holding these teeth. These teeth are loose.

When sufficient bone has been lost, the tooth loosens. When a tooth loosens, the destruction of bone around it may accelerate.

Finally, when deprived of most of the supporting bone, the tooth becomes so loose that it either falls out or must be removed.

NATURAL RESISTANCE OR SUSCEPTIBILITY TO PERIODONTAL DISEASES

Very few people are totally *resistant* to periodontal diseases. Most are quite *susceptible*.

However, most people have a varying resistance to these diseases at different times in their lives. For example, a person's resistance may be normal for years. Then resistance temporarily diminishes and periodontal disease appears, or disease that was under control flares up.

While periodontal diseases cannot be cured, in most cases you and your dentist together can slow down or arrest the disease. For the majority of people, tooth loss can be prevented.

THE PERIODONTAL EXAMINATION

You cannot accurately diagnose periodontal diseases yourself:

• They most often start between back teeth where you can't see them.

• They will almost always be painless.

• There is usually no "pink toothbrush" (bleeding) to warn you.

Therefore, even if you never have cavities, and your mouth feels fine, *go for regular dental checkups*. Your dentist and hygienist can spot disease early, when it is the easiest—and least costly—to treat. This early detection is possible only with a measuring instrument called the *periodontal probe*. This device can find periodontal diseases long before they show up on x-rays.

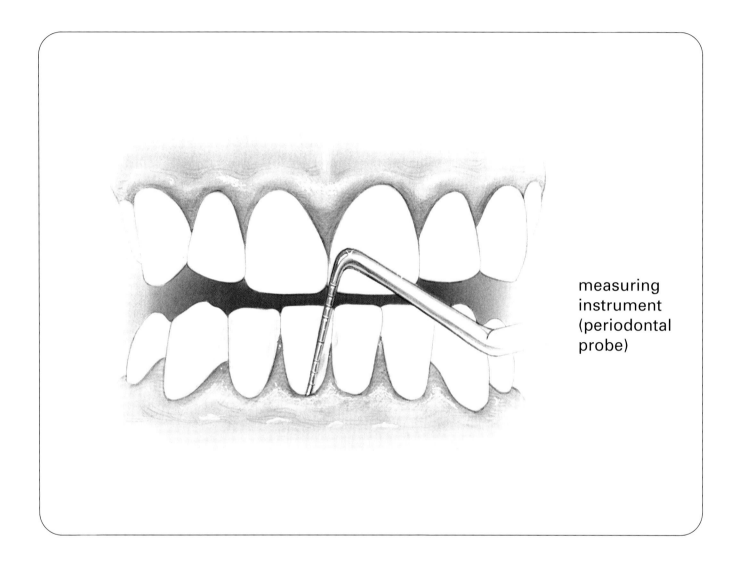

measuring
instrument
(periodontal
probe)

The dentist or dental hygienist will gently examine for hidden areas of disease *(pockets)*.

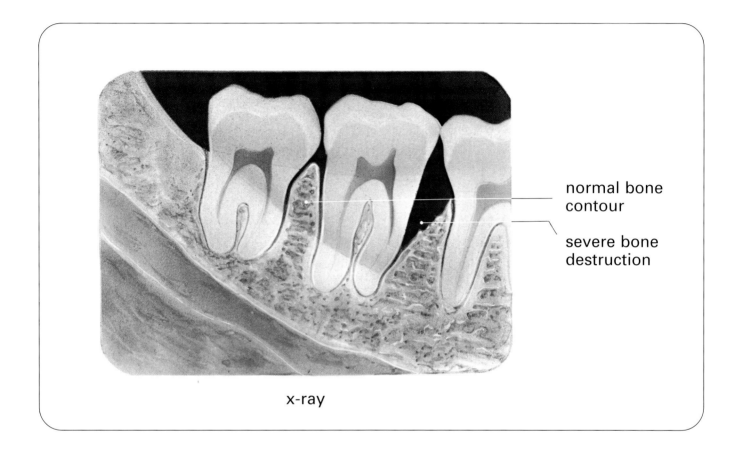

normal bone
contour

severe bone
destruction

x-ray

Your dentist will also need a complete set of x-rays to help in diagnosis and treatment planning.

THE SPECIALIST

If you have a periodontal problem that does not respond to routine care, or if you have advanced disease, you may need to see a *periodontist*.

A periodontist is a specialist in the care of the gums and supporting bone. He has years of extra schooling and experience that permit him to use special techniques to treat more difficult or more advanced periodontal problems.

CONCLUSIONS OF PART I

1. Periodontal diseases are infections.

2. The primary cause of these infections is plaque, a sticky colony of living bacteria. If left on the teeth, plaque forms calculus (tartar), which you cannot safely remove at home.

3. Millions of people have some type of periodontal disease, but most do not realize they have the problem.

4. There are two stages of periodontal diseases:
   a. *Gingivitis*, an infection of the gum.
   b. *Periodontitis* (pyorrhea), an infection that involves the supporting bone.

5. See your dentist on a regular basis, even if you think nothing is wrong. Only a professional can diagnose periodontal diseases in their earliest stages, when they are the easiest—and least costly—to treat. Loss of all your teeth from periodontal diseases is *not* inevitable. You and your dentist, working together, can see to that.

PART II

PART II will tell you, step by step, how periodontal diseases cause the loss of a tooth.

First let's look at some important relationships between the teeth, the gums, and the bone.

The teeth within the square opposite will appear in the diagrams that follow.

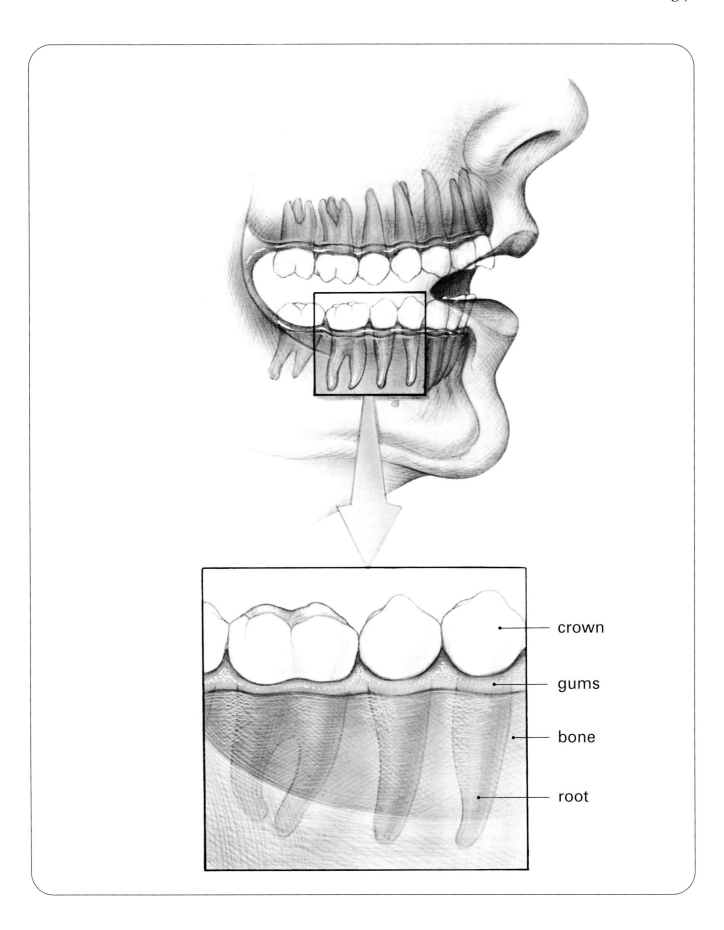

crown

gums

bone

root

This drawing shows what is beneath the surface.

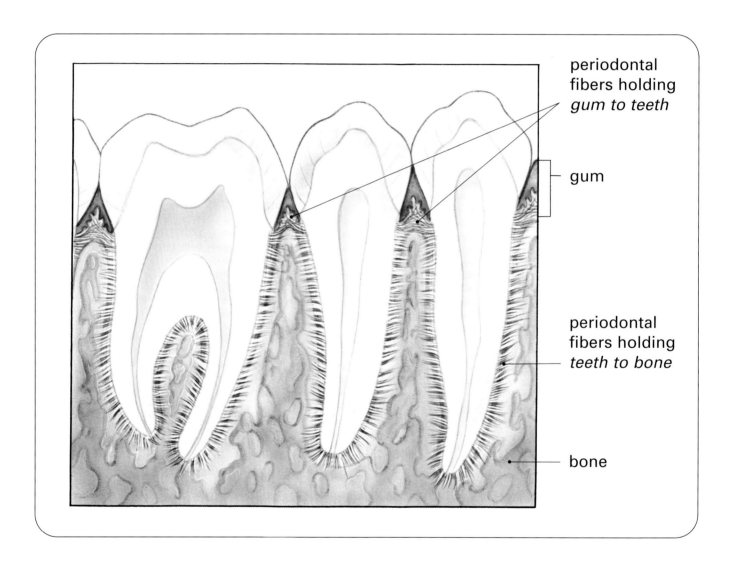

periodontal fibers holding *gum to teeth*

gum

periodontal fibers holding *teeth to bone*

bone

Many thousands of fibers, called *periodontal fibers*, go from their origins on the roots of the teeth into the gums or the surrounding bone.

Those *fibers that enter the gums* pull the gums into a tight collar around the necks of the teeth.

The great mass of *fibers that go from the roots into the bone* attach the teeth to the bone.

Some people mistakenly believe that teeth are "in the gums." Not so. Teeth are in bone. The gums are a protective covering over this bone. In a healthy mouth, the gums hug the teeth like tight collars to prevent bacteria and food debris from invading the bone. Simply put, the gums protect the bone, and the bone holds the teeth.

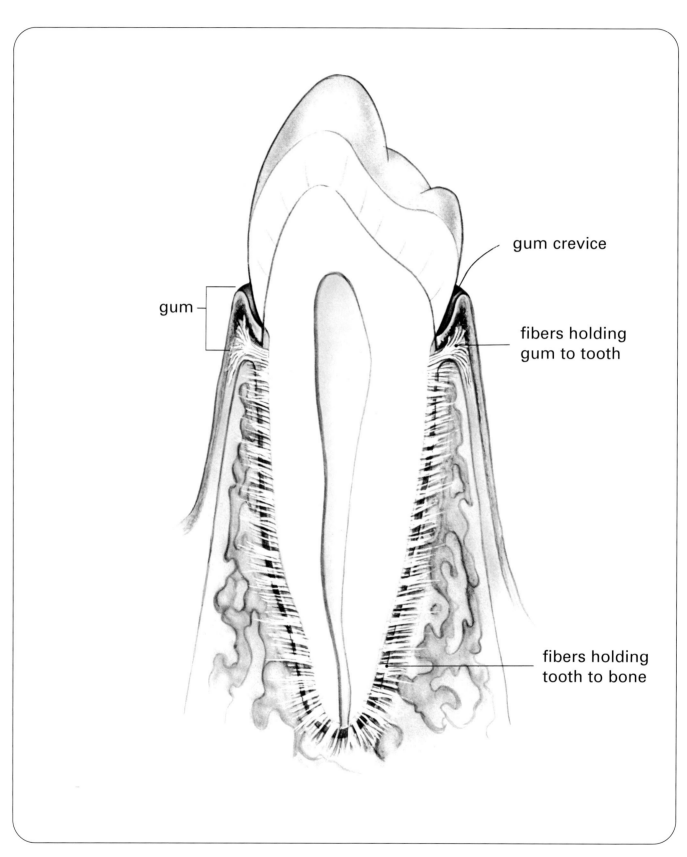

gum crevice

gum

fibers holding
gum to tooth

fibers holding
tooth to bone

This isolated tooth is enlarged nine times the normal size.

The fibers going from the root into the gum pull the gum tightly against the crown. There is a small crevice between the gum and tooth that you don't see when you look in your mouth. This area, where the gum lies against the crown, has been called the *gum crevice* (or *sulcus*).

The depth of this crevice is of major importance.

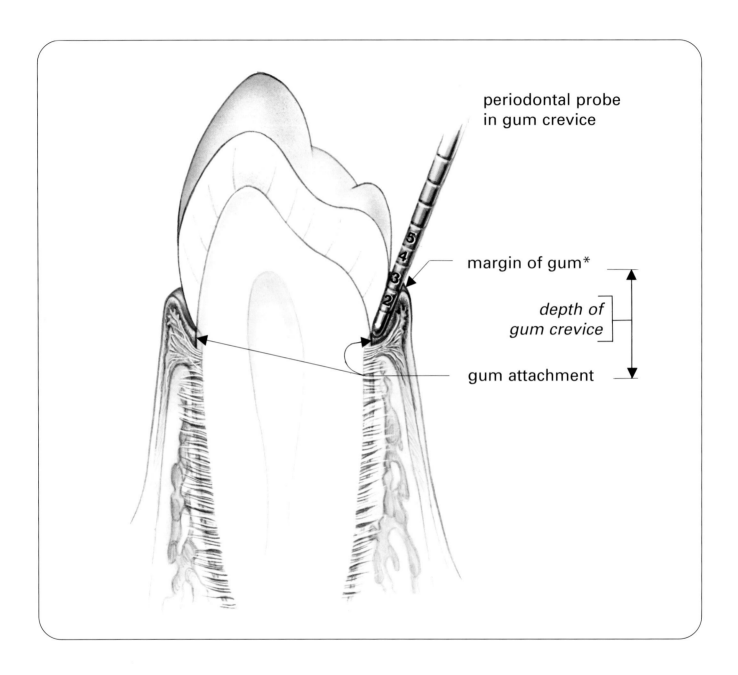

periodontal probe
in gum crevice

margin of gum*

depth of
gum crevice

gum attachment

We have placed a periodontal probe gently to the bottom of the crevice to measure its depth. The *attachment of the gum* limits how far the instrument can go.

*The *margin* of the gum is its upper edge.

The markings on the periodontal probe are 1 mm apart. (An actual millimeter is the distance between these two lines ══.)

Normal crevices measure 1 to 3 mm deep. The crevice in this drawing is 2 mm deep.

The next few pages will help you to understand how periodontal diseases actually progress.

Keep in mind as you read that you and your dentist can prevent periodontal diseases. Even if disease has started, you and your dentist together can treat it. Most people do not have to lose their teeth.

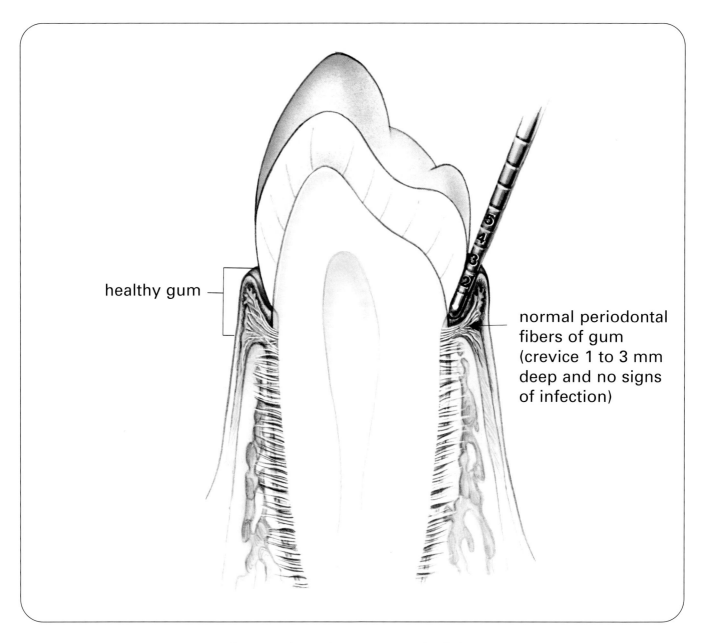

healthy gum

normal periodontal
fibers of gum
(crevice 1 to 3 mm
deep and no signs
of infection)

NORMAL AND HEALTHY

Periodontal fibers hold the normal gum tightly against the tooth.

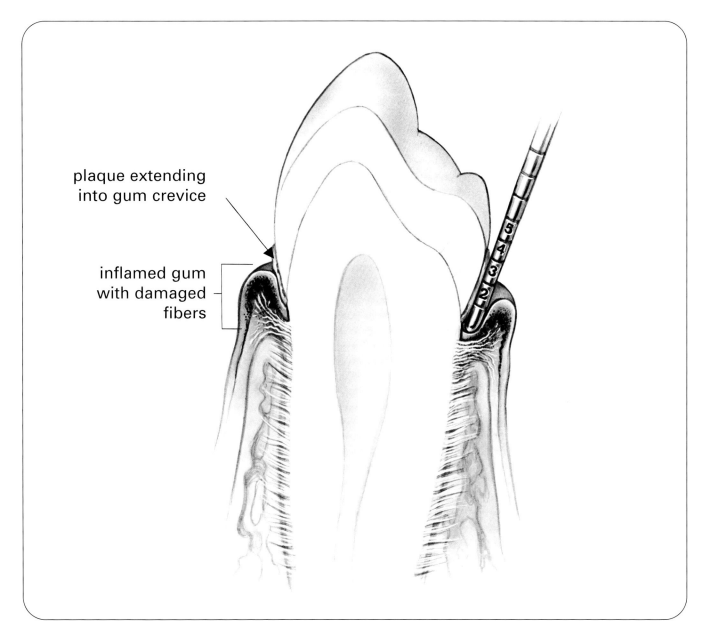

plaque extending
into gum crevice

inflamed gum
with damaged
fibers

STAGE ONE OF DISEASE: GINGIVITIS

Plaque has caused infection. The gum usually looks normal. Often, only your dentist can discover disease at this stage. Inflammation damages the periodontal fibers that hold the gum tightly against the tooth. This allows plaque to enter deeper into the gum crevice, where it can do even more damage.

Professional treatment and good personal home care at this earliest stage can usually arrest the disease. The gums restore themselves to full health, with no permanent damage.

STAGE TWO:
EARLY PERIODONTITIS (EARLY BONE LOSS)

If plaque irritation persists, it causes the *attachment of the gum to move down the root*. This "creeping" of the gum attachment makes the crevice deeper.

A crevice more than 3 mm deep is considered a *pocket*. Pockets are very hard to keep clean. They are impossible to keep clean once calculus has formed within them. The toxins from the plaque in the pocket shown opposite have also destroyed some adjacent bone.

Professional treatment plus good home care can slow or stop the progress of disease at this stage.

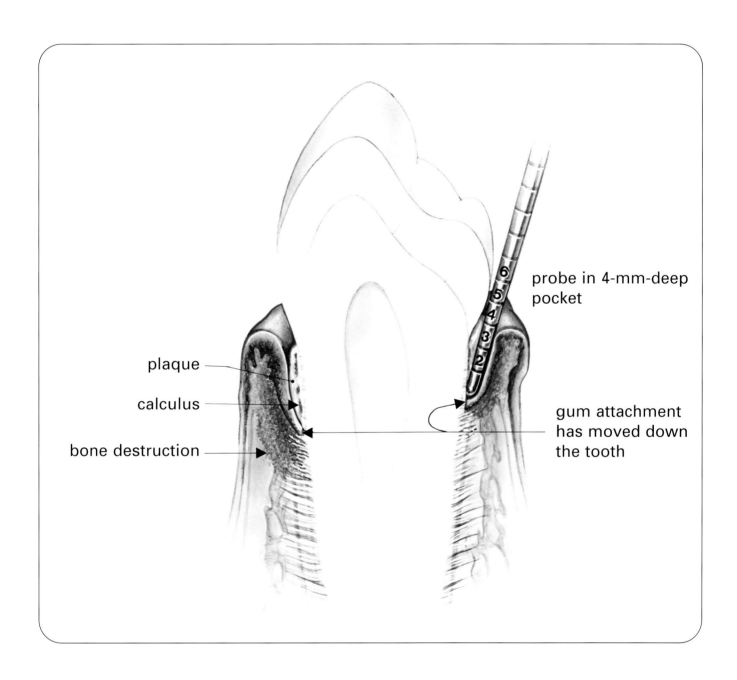

plaque

calculus

bone destruction

probe in 4-mm-deep pocket

gum attachment has moved down the tooth

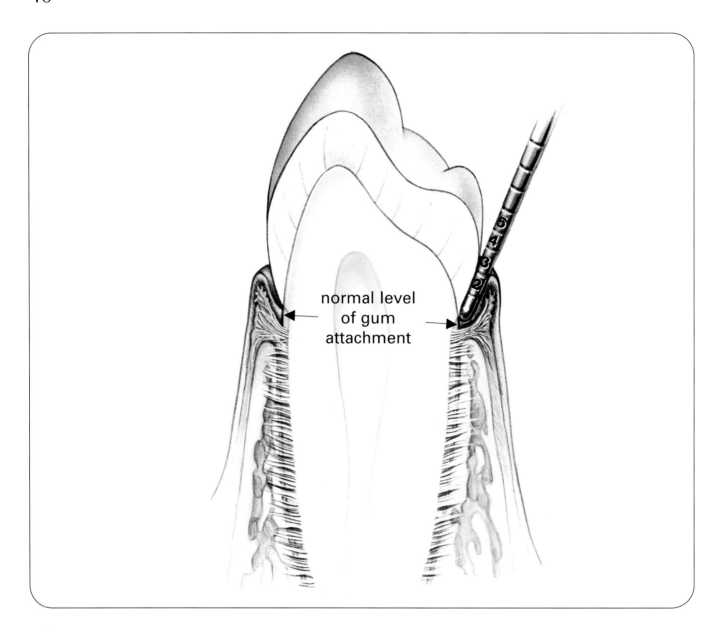

normal level
of gum
attachment

NORMAL AND HEALTHY

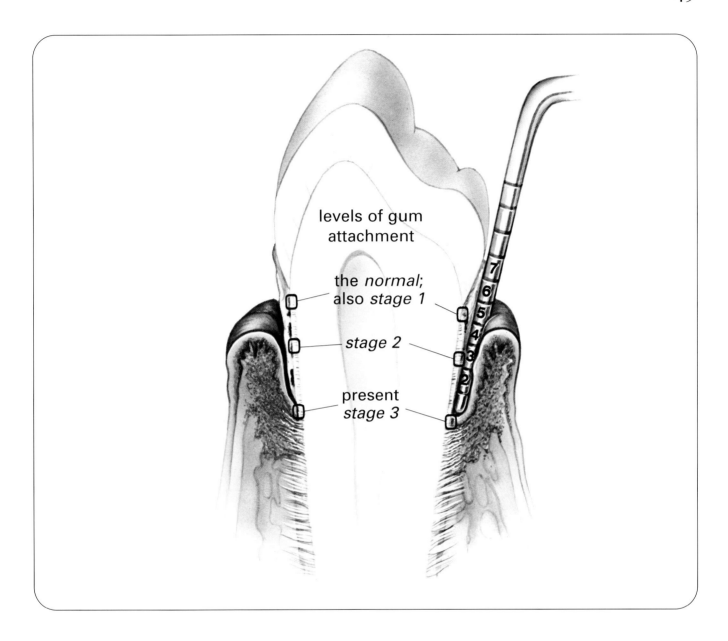

levels of gum attachment

the *normal;* also *stage 1*

stage 2

present *stage 3*

STAGE THREE:
MODERATE PERIODONTITIS (MODERATE BONE LOSS)

Continuing infection has caused the loss of up to one third of bone support, as the gum attachment has crept further down the root. Pockets depths usually range from 5 to 6 mm. Again, professional treatment plus good home care can stop the progress of disease at this stage.

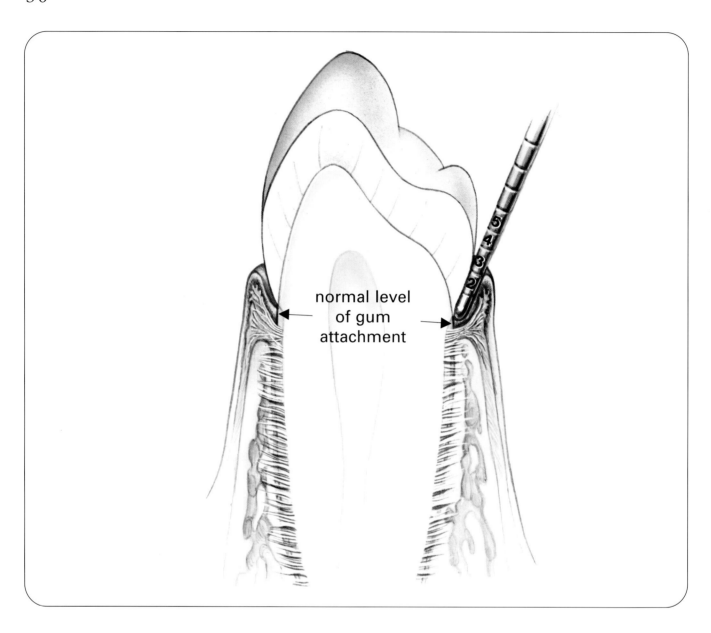

normal level
of gum
attachment

NORMAL AND HEALTHY

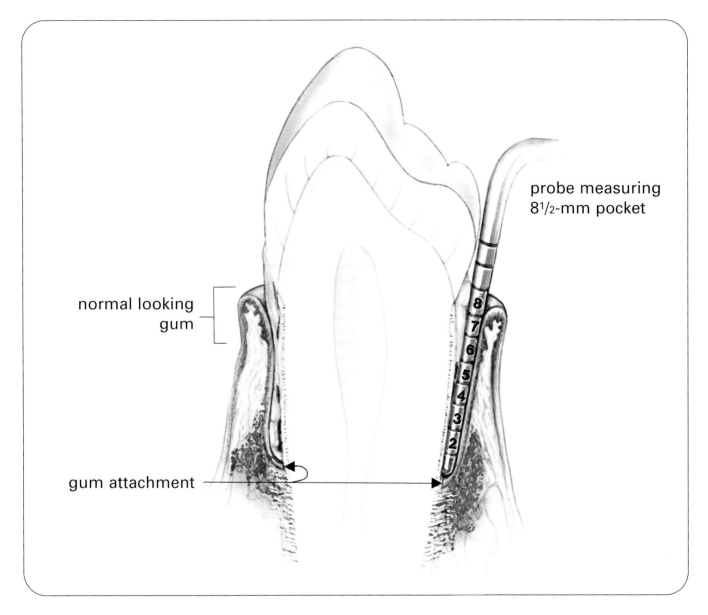

normal looking gum

probe measuring 8½-mm pocket

gum attachment

STAGE FOUR:
SEVERE PERIODONTITIS (ADVANCED BONE LOSS)

Half or more of the original bone holding the tooth has been lost and pockets usually are 7 mm or deeper. The margin of the gum may withdraw down the root. This recession of the gums exposes part of the root and makes the tooth look longer.

Even in this advanced stage of periodontal disease, professional treatment and proper home care usually help considerably. In some cases it is possible to replace lost bone by using advanced surgical techniques.

The diagram on the opposite page dramatically shows how much bone loss and gum recession have taken place at STAGE FOUR.

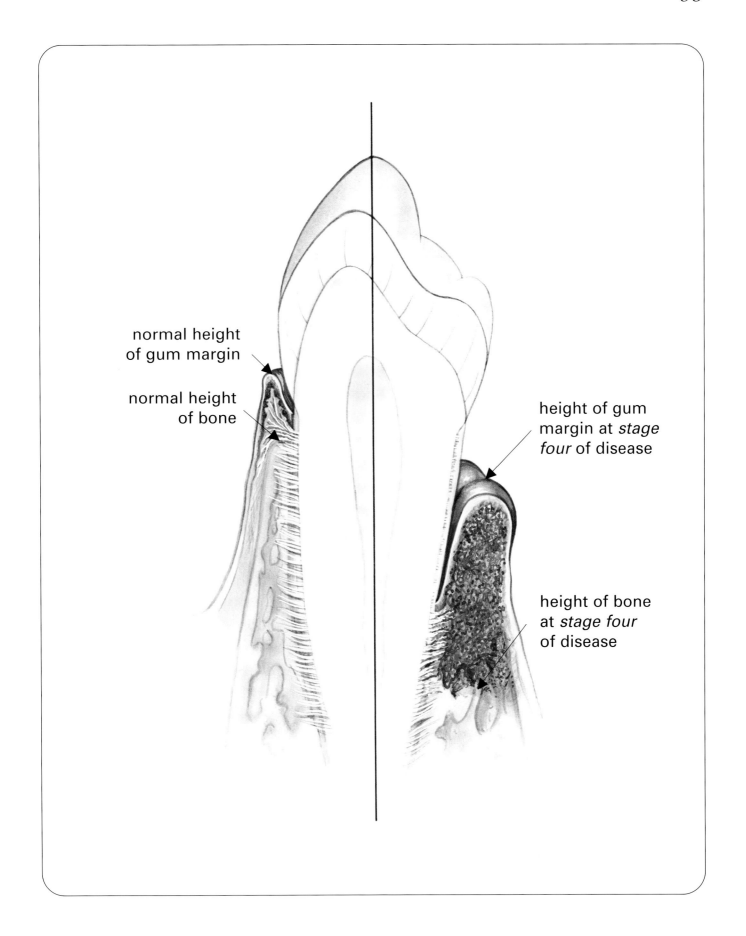

normal height
of gum margin

normal height
of bone

height of gum
margin at *stage
four* of disease

height of bone
at *stage four*
of disease

THE RESULTS OF UNTREATED PERIODONTITIS

Now it is too late for any treatment. Not enough bone remains, and the inflammation surrounds the entire root end. The tooth is very loose. If your dentist does not extract the tooth, it will eventually fall out.

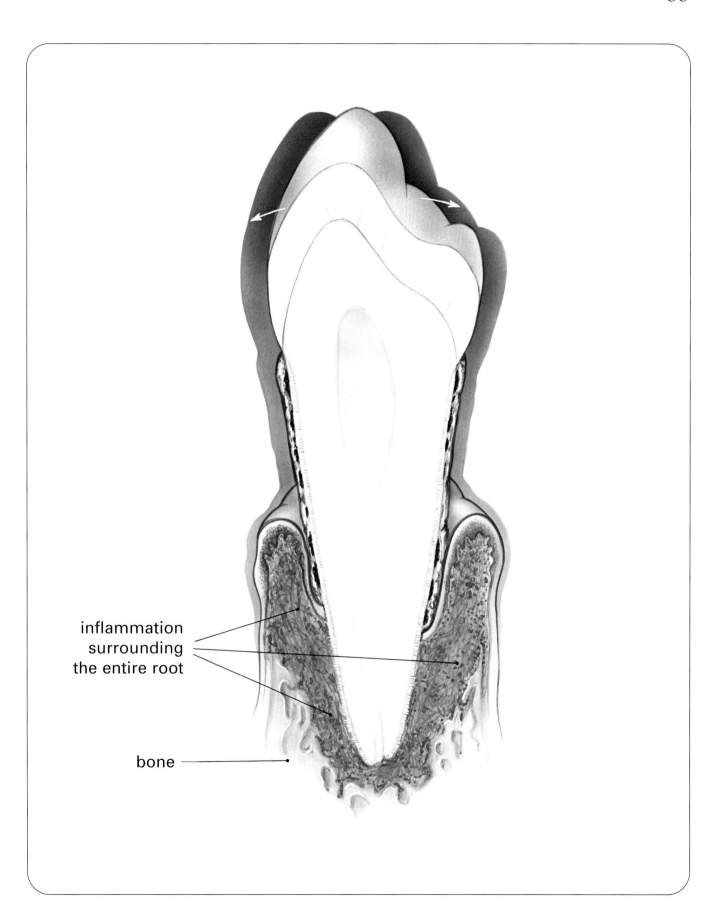

inflammation surrounding the entire root

bone

CONCLUSIONS OF PART II

Plaque bacteria produce the *toxins* that cause the infections of periodontal diseases.

If untreated, periodontal diseases often cause *bone loss*.

If periodontal disease destroys enough of the bone supporting a tooth, the tooth will be lost.

Periodontal diseases need not happen:

• Brush and floss properly to remove all the plaque.

• Get regular periodontal examinations, including periodontal probings.

• Follow through on any necessary treatment.

PART III

PART III will explain how your dental professional, with your cooperation, can treat periodontal diseases to reduce the chance of tooth loss.

Most treatment involves:

1. Personal oral hygiene
2. Professional removal of plaque and calculus
3. Professional assessment of the "bite"
4. Professional maintenance

1. PERSONAL ORAL HYGIENE

One of the most important things a dental professional will do is *take the time to teach you proper flossing and brushing*. Few people do it correctly without instruction. The cost of *not* learning to floss and brush the right way could be the loss of your teeth.

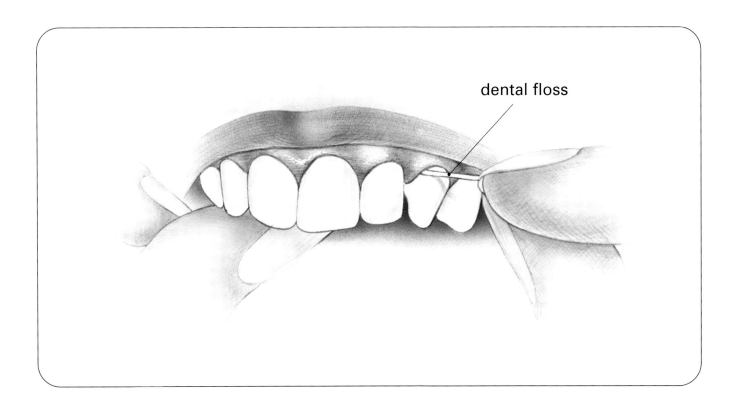

It is important to floss every day.

Dental floss removes the plaque from between the teeth, where the toothbrush can't reach.

If you brush but don't floss, you are doing only *half* the job.

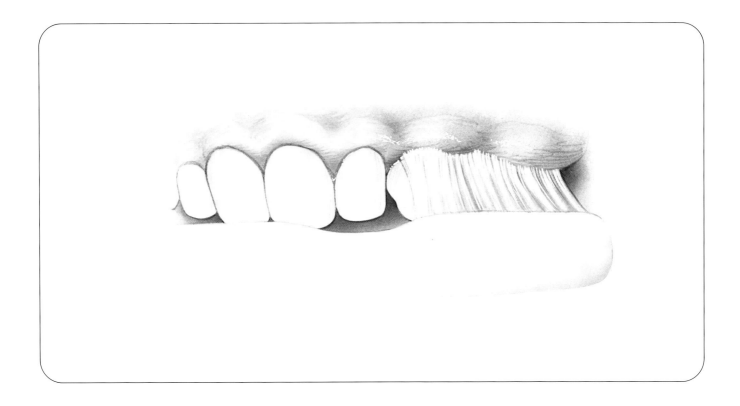

It is important to brush correctly every day.

Toothbrush bristles remove the plaque from exposed surfaces of the teeth. It is the tips of the bristles of a toothbrush that do the work. Therefore, when the bristles have bent over or curled from use, replace your brush.

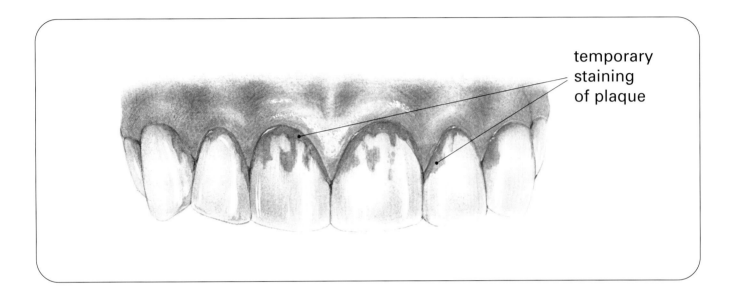

temporary
staining
of plaque

Drugstores sell inexpensive *disclosing tablets* that contain a harmless vegetable dye. You should occasionally dissolve one in your mouth after flossing and brushing. It will temporarily stain any plaque you have missed, showing you areas where you must make a special effort to clean more thoroughly.

2. PROFESSIONAL REMOVAL OF PLAQUE AND CALCULUS

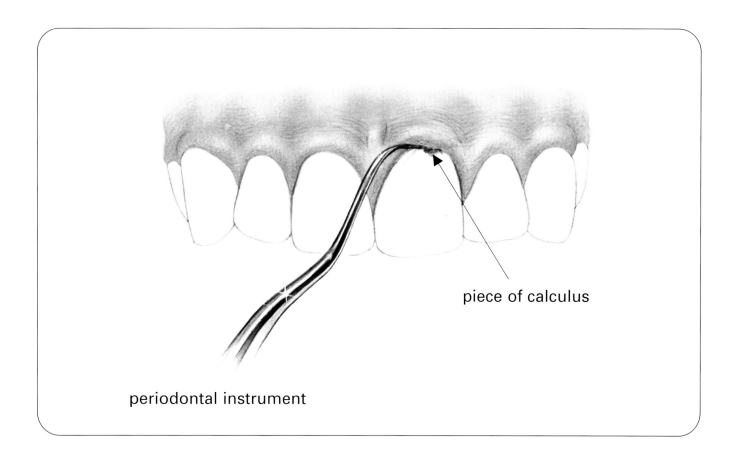

piece of calculus

periodontal instrument

Your dentist or dental hygienist will gently remove the calculus above and below the gum. In some cases of moderate and severe periodontitis, it may be necessary to lift the gum back to remove as much calculus as possible or to attempt to regrow lost bone.

Your dentist will check any restorations for correct *shape and fit*. Fillings and crowns that no longer fit will trap bacteria and food debris. This can cause severe periodontal problems. Have such fillings or crowns repaired or replaced.

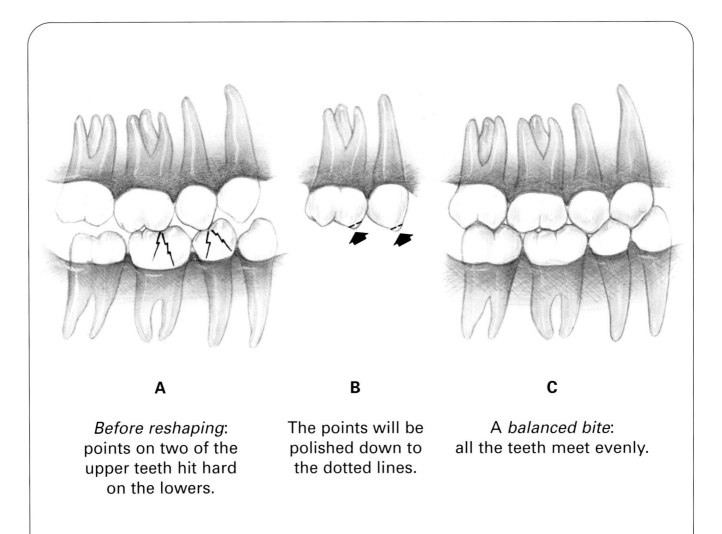

A

Before reshaping: points on two of the upper teeth hit hard on the lowers.

B

The points will be polished down to the dotted lines.

C

A *balanced bite*: all the teeth meet evenly.

3. PROFESSIONAL ASSESSMENT OF THE "BITE"

A *balanced bite* (one where the teeth meet evenly during chewing) is important for many reasons, but it can be crucial when periodontal inflammation is being treated. Too much force on a tooth with periodontal disease can cause bone loss to accelerate.

Your dentist may inspect the way your upper and lower teeth come together (the "bite") to see if the forces of chewing are evenly distributed among all the teeth. If you are chewing on some teeth harder than on others, he may gently reshape the biting surfaces of these teeth until they meet evenly.

4. PROFESSIONAL MAINTENANCE

It is very common for periodontitis to recur. Patients should have regular checkups to catch recurrence early, before silent damage occurs. Many patients with periodontitis will have to get checkups, usually accompanied by a professional tooth cleaning, every 3 months. These checkups, which catch disease in its early stages, will prevent suffering, save money, and provide the best chance against tooth loss.

CONCLUSIONS OF PART III

Prevention and treatment of periodontal diseases involves the combined efforts of you, your dentist (or periodontal specialist), and the personnel who clean your teeth.

They will remove plaque and calculus that may have formed despite your best efforts at home care.

They will check for factors that contribute to periodontitis, such as defective fillings or crowns or a bad bite.

They will check on your brushing and flossing techniques.

They will provide regular maintenance care after initial treatment of periodontitis.

But professional care is only half the battle in preventing—or curing—periodontal diseases. The *essential* other half depends on you to brush and floss every day.

The good news is, with care, your teeth can last a lifetime.